I0488980

11 Essential Probiotic Rich Foods To Change Your Life

Discover How To Naturally Cure Diseases, Fight Infections And Improve Your Digestive System

Joseph J. Miller

© 2015

Disclaimer

This book is not intended as a substitute for the medical advice of physicians. The reader should regularly consult a physician in matters relating to his/her health and particularly with respect to any symptoms that may require diagnosis or medical attention.

Table of Contents

Introduction

Nutrition plays a huge role in every human being's quality of health. You are not an exception to the rule. What you eat or do not eat will affect you externally and internally regardless of what stage you are in life. Healthy nutrition can protect an unborn child from disease and it can reverse aging in a mature adult.

There is growing awareness about the way to maintain good health, particularly through better nutrition. People are increasingly sourcing and opting for holistic and alternative health methods to cope with disease and promote longevity. With modern technology, obtaining information about nutritional benefits of certain kinds of food is easy to obtain from all over the world. Again, groundbreaking innovation in science has helped us validate what foods are actually beneficial and what is not.

Over the centuries man has existed, there has been a need to preserve and store food in order to make it available during seasons they were not accessible. Roasting, blending, wrapping in leaves, storing in containers made of clay, metal and later, glass has evolved today into domestic preservation techniques like refrigeration and commercial preservation methods like pasteurization and facilities like commercial silos.

The same science through which modern preservation techniques emanated is reviewing prehistoric storage techniques and diets. Scientists are beginning to discover that certain foods preserved in certain kinds of ways, particularly through fermenting, were not only available when out of season, but provided certain nutrients that were very beneficial to our overall health. One of such nutrients is a special live bacterium previously unpopular and rarely talked about known as probiotics.

Previously, the role of probiotics in the human body was not getting the attention it truly deserved. Now, it is slowly increasing and even soaring in popularity. Let us go further to discuss probiotics in detail.

What 'EXACTLY' are Probiotics

The word 'Probiotic' comes from the combination of two Latin words: 'pro' which means 'for' and 'biotic' an adjective derived from the word 'bios' which means 'life'. Hence 'probiotic' literally means 'for life'. They are live microorganisms (yeasts or bacteria) which can confer numerous health benefits when consumed in adequate quantities and regular intervals. In simpler terms, they are healthy bacteria.

To get a better understanding of what probiotics are, we need to understand that there is a high level of bacteria in the body of every human being. In fact, each one of us usually has ten to twenty times more bacteria in our body. The bacteria in our body actually outnumber the number of cells in our body. There are actually about 400 different types of microorganisms that we are host to and about 85% are very crucial in maintaining our health.[1] Different strains of probiotics deliver specific health benefits. We are estimated to host an amount of bacteria equivalent to the total number of human beings that have ever lived on the planet.

The natural balance of good and bad bacteria does several things for our bodies. First, they form a barrier in our abdomen to ensure that beneficial nutrients are absorbed and retained for use within the body. They also keep toxic substances out of the body. Overall, the presence of probiotics helps us optimize our intestinal function by establishing a balance in the level of beneficial microorganisms within our intestinal walls thereby promoting good health.

Why Do We Need Probiotics

Our modern day diets are nutritionally deficient and overloaded with sugar, hydrogenated fats, salt, refined carbohydrates, chemical preservatives and many other unhealthy components. They are technically fillers and hardly deliver any health benefits to our system.

Although probiotics are present within our bodies, they need to be reinforced regularly or they will deplete and deliver lesser benefits. The role of these bacteria cannot be ignored. Good bacteria fight bad bacteria in order to ward off disease hence boost our immunity. Put in another way, they are a first line defense for fighting any unwanted invasion into our bodies.

Probiotics also aid in several aspects of digestion by helping us break down food, adequately extract beneficial nutrients. Scientists and medical personnel increasingly believe that we probably need to take probiotics the same way we take vitamins. From small health problems like common cold to significant health challenges like cancer, intake of probiotics will deliver some relief to the body.

To ensure that we have enough levels of probiotics in our systems to regulate our health we need to 'refuel' with probiotic rich foods regularly. A healthy diet that is rich in probiotics can slow down and even reverse the effects of disease in the human body.

Probiotics convey a lot of innumerable benefits to our bodies that cannot be ignored.

Probiotics & Gastrointestinal Function

Digestive problems like indigestion, diarrhea and constipation are so common and accepted as 'normal' by most of us on the planet. An estimated 95 million of American suffer from Gastro Intestinal dysfunction.[2] This is about thirty percent of the population. Irritable Bowel Syndrome better known as IBS is one of the top ten reasons for visiting a doctor in the United States. About $105 billion US dollar is spent on medical treatments for GI conditions in the United States every year.

Our gastrointestinal system is primarily responsible for approximately 80% of the health of the immune system. Improving your gut health has been scientifically proved to affect your total health and wellbeing.

Probiotics offer some of the most important solutions for dealing with digestive health issues, doing a number of specific things in the gut. Acidophilus and other probiotics secrete antibacterial, antifungal and antiviral chemicals in the gut. Acidophilus also creates an acidic microenvironment which helps us increase our absorption of iron and other beneficial minerals. They also form a protective physical wall or lining to ward of invasion of bacteria and yeast.

Intake of probiotic rich foods has been shown to reduce the symptoms of inflammatory bowel disease, diarrhea and allergies to certain foods. Some research is examining their prohibitive effects on colorectal cancer.[3]

In summary, probiotics inhibit the growth of harmful bacteria in our gut that trigger off stress during digestion, improve the digestion and absorption of trace minerals like calcium and enhance our overall metabolism.

Probiotics & Your Immune System

A healthy gut is usually has a lot of healthy bacteria. These bacteria are 'at war' with the unhealthy bacteria also present in the gut. Feeding them constantly with probiotics food boosts your allies i.e. the healthy bacteria, with what they need to defend you. Boosting the healthy bacteria in your gut strengthens about 80% of your body's total immune system's health.

There is one thing we all have to know about the harmful micro-organisms in our body. We live in a world where healthy eating habits isn't practiced enough. Fast, cheap, processed, sugary, genetically modified foods are at available at the snap of a finger. Most of these foods do not have any significant healthy nutritional content in them. And apart from fats, preservatives, carcinogenic contents in processed foods, one major dangerous substance they contain is sugar.

Most of this sugar is hidden through deceptive labelling. Words like 'Fructose', 'Sweeteners', 'Sucrose' and many more are used to deceive us that our foods do not contain sugar when the truth is that they are loaded with it and causing serious problems to our health. Many diseases have links to high sugar intake. Diabetes is an obvious outcome of excess intake of sugar. When the body can no longer metabolize sugar, it is converted and stored as fat which leads to obesity. Cancer cells feed on sugar.

The unhealthy bacteria in our gut thrive and multiply vigorously when we eat foods containing sugar. Once they multiply and outnumber the good bacteria, they weaken our immune system leaving us open to disease infection. The natural way to reverse the situation is to increase our intake of probiotic rich foods so they can repair our immune systems. Taking probiotic rich foods constantly also helps us ward off sickness and remain healthy. Probiotics are a natural defense system for our bodies.

Probiotics & Brain Function

Our mind and even our mood are closely linked to how healthy our gut is. This is because the larger bulk of the serotonin used up by the brain, is produced in the gut.

The quality of health in our gut will affect the output of our mind, mood and overall mental health. The gut actually is the second brain. When people say 'gut feeling', they might just be right after all. The brain is interconnected to our body's organ systems.

Probiotic bacteria have been shown to promote the growth and development of neurons, stimulate memory and learning, guide changes in our mood, change our digestive patterns and even change the pattern of genetic expression. (Grossman, 2015)

Immune abnormalities affect the brain and can lead to neurological disorders. Though the study of gut flora is complex, researchers are immersed in several studies to determine how it can be beneficial to treating diseases like Alzheimer's, Parkinson's, autism and multiple sclerosis.

Other Health Benefits of Probiotics

Apart from digestive health, there are several other benefits that stem from taking probiotics. These include:

- They reduce infections like candida and vaginal yeast.
- They help in managing blood pressure
- They can help lower cholesterol
- The can help lactose intolerant people digest lactose
- They can decrease dental caries microbes which may be present in the mouth
- They help fight allergies
- They help with reducing inflammation
- They help with skin rejuvenation and dealing with certain skin conditions like dermatitis and eczema.
- They help increase metabolism as well as our natural flora after we take prescription medication.[4]

The numerous benefits of probiotics cannot be fully mentioned and there is still a lot of on-going research to unveil more about them. We cannot do wrong by increasing this life giving microorganisms in our diet.

Foods Rich In Probiotics

A lot of people take probiotic supplements. While nutritional supplements may deliver the some benefits, the dosage and efficacy of probiotics from supplements are not guaranteed. A study done on 55 different brands of probiotic supplements discovered that only 13% of them actually delivered the quantity of probiotics on the packaging. Moreover, it is not always guaranteed that the preservation process will not damage the probiotics contained in the supplements. Probiotics are particularly more delicate than most other nutrients because they are 'alive' i.e. 'living microorganisms'. They are best obtained through food.

Most foods containing probiotics are 'cultures'. These foods are derived from a primary food source which is fermented in other to get the benefit of probiotics from the end product. Fermenting food is not a modern technique. In ancient times, foods were fermented either to preserve them or to derive a new food or condiment from them.

Fermentation breaks down the molecules of a food into a more basic form: bacteria convert carbohydrates to lactic acid and yeast turn sugar into alcohol. Also, some people erroneously believe that probiotics are only available through dairy products and this is untrue. There are non-dairy sources of probiotics and these are great for lactose intolerant people.

Any food source we decide to take to increase our dose of probiotics has to be natural or organic. Many food preservation processes destroy probiotics. Avoid processed foods particularly those which have been pasteurized. They will not deliver adequate quantity or quality of probiotics. It is not really hard to find at least one food which can supply your body with a healthy dose of probiotics no matter what part of the planet you live. Let us look at some of the foods that are rich in probiotics.

1. Live, Cultured Yogurt

Yogurt always tops the charts as the first food to go for when looking for a rich source of probiotics. The problem with yogurt is that most commercial available yogurt is pasteurized as well as packed full with sugar and preservatives and because of this, they do not contain any probiotics at all.

Even when you resort to more organic brands and unsweetened varieties like Greek yogurt, not every brand is the same. Some higher quality brands might even deliver fewer probiotics than brands perceived to be lower.

Natural, organic, unprocessed yogurt is best for a reasonable supply of probiotics. The refined, sweetened and fancy packaged yogurts do not have any significant probiotic activity/content. Homemade, unprocessed yoghurt has very high probiotic content. Yogurt from goat milk is said to particularly have a rich probiotic level.

Knowledge of what to look out for in the product label is important in order to get a product that truly delivers a good amount of probiotics. Labels that have phrases like 'live and active cultures' might have a higher dose of probiotic content. And a lot of brands will further list the names of the probiotics the yogurt might contain. These might be names like bifidus regularis, S.Thermophilus, bifidobacterium L.Bulgaricus, etc.[5] Checking the label will ensure you get value for your money. Avoid any products with high fructose, corn syrup, sugar, sweeteners, artificial flavors, additives and artificial flavors. The more basic, organic and unflavored the yogurt is, then the more likely it is it will have a higher quantity of probiotic.

Several studies have been conducted and they found that consumption of yogurt was indeed beneficial particularly to digestive health (Irritable Bowel Syndrome[6] (IBS) and diarrhea), upper respiratory illnesses and even brain health. The only clause is that regular and not occasional consumption is required before any significant changes can be noticed.

In addition to probiotics, consuming yogurt will also deliver a good dose of animal protein as well as other beneficial nutrients like vitamins and minerals. People who are lactose intolerant can also consume yogurt.

Yogurt is great because it can be consumed without further processing as well as added to other treats, desserts and smoothies. However, if yogurt were heated before use, the probiotic content would be destroyed by heat. It is best eaten cold or at most, room temperature.

2. Kefir

Kefir (also known as keefir or kephir) is soaring in popularity amongst health food enthusiasts all around the world for very good reasons. It is a fermented drink made by adding kefir grains to goat or cow milk and leaving it for about 24 to 48 hours to ferment. During this time, the lactic bacteria in the kefir seeds break down the lactose in the milk into lactic acid. After this, the milk is strained and the gel-like kefir grains (which look similar to cauliflower) can be reused to ferment more milk into kefir. The strained milk tastes like sour yoghurt but has a thinner consistency.

The making of the kefir grains has remained a mystery with several theories or stories trying to offer an explanation to how they originated. In ancient times, they were simply said to be food from the gods. One theory says that it came from sheep mouth or intestinal bacteria. Another account is that shepherds who carried milk in leather wineskin pouches frequently discovered that it would occasionally ferment into an effervescent drink.[7] Another legend from the Caucasian mountains has it that it was a gift from the Islamic prophet Mohammed who taught his followers how to use it and forbade from divulging the secret of its preparation to anyone hence they are known as 'grains of the prophet'. The mystery surrounding how kefir is made is a blessing in disguise because scientist have still not uncovered it and this makes kefir one of the unadulterated, authentic foods in the world.

Not only is kefir rich in nutrients, it also has a high amount of probiotics. Kefir grains contain about 30 – 35 different strains of yeast and bacteria which make it a more potent in probiotics than yoghurt. There is even a specific probiotic known as lactobacillus kefir which is only found in kefir.

One great advantage kefir has is that it is well tolerated by people who are lactose intolerant[8]. Apart from this, kefir is very versatile. It can also be made with non-dairy liquids like fruit juice or coconut water. A great tip is to make your own kefir drink. It is very simple to make. The commercially available kefir is usually not fermented long enough and pasteurization significantly reduced the probiotics in the drink.[9] And when making kefir, use the milk from grass fed cows or goats milk to get the best delivery of probiotics in the drink.

Some users also advice that kefir should be introduced into your diet in small quantities and consumption can be increased as time goes on. Ingesting large quantities from the start might cause undesirable reactions.

3. Miso

For over 2,500 years, from ancient China to Japan and now, miso has been a major staple. It is a savory and flavor-packed paste which can be used as a condiment in soup and is said to have anti-aging benefits and also neutralize effects of smoking, radiation and air pollution in the human body.

Miso itself is a paste or a culture made by combining cooked, ground soybeans, [10] koji, salt and water into a paste which is then molded into balls and fermenting them in a container for up to six months to as much as two or three years.[11] The longer miso is fermented, the higher the quality of the final product in addition to having a richer, more complex and flavor. The making of miso is a craft that has been perfected by the Japanese.

It would be necessary to explain what koji is. Koji is sometimes mistaken by people that are not Japanese as yeast, but it is actually a mold with sweet fragrance made with cooked rice[12]which is infused with a fermentation culture widely available in Japan known as aspergillus oryzae. So in an actual sense, koji is a fermentation starter. Koji is used in a wide range of Japanese dishes like soy sauce, sake, mirin, pickles and rice vinegar.

Miso paste is a versatile seasoning. Apart from soups, it can be used in sauces for fish or meat and even for homemade salad dressing. One caution about using miso is to remember that it is usually high in salt. Our recommended daily intake of sodium is 2,400 milligrams and an average teaspoon of miso contains approximately 250 grams of salt.[13] You probably would need to completely forgo or tone down the amount of salt in your dish or use miso in moderate quantities. People who are allergic to soya bean should also avoid miso.

The fermentation process of the miso along with the infusion of koji ensures that miso delivers a good dosage of probiotics. It is important to add miso at the end of any cooking process so that the heat from cooking will not destroy the beneficial probiotics it contains. Unpasteurized miso is best and storing in an airtight container kept in the refrigerator is the best way to preserve miso.

4. Sauerkraut

Some people have a hard time digesting cabbage and sauerkraut is a great alternative for them. Sauerkraut is also a great source of probiotics for people who are lactose intolerant to get probiotics in their diet. Again, just like most other probiotic food sources, commercially sold sauerkraut is usually preserved through pasteurization so it does not deliver any probiotic nutrients. Homemade sauerkraut is best.

Sauerkraut simply means 'sour cabbage' in German. It is a sort of 'pickled cabbage' made by cutting, bruising and pressing or squeezing cabbage with some salt[14] to extract its water or juice, then storing in a jar with the juice extracted where it is left to ferment for about twelve days up to three months. When ready for consumption, the cabbage changes color from green to pale yellow.

Sauerkraut is usually eaten hot or cold but if you desire to get the probiotics from it, then it is best eaten cold as heat destroys the probiotic content. There are several ways to eat sauerkraut in cold dishes. Examples are including it as filling in hot dogs or sandwiches, adding it to cold salads, potato dishes, eggs, fish, meat or serving it as a condiment to the main meal. Some people add sauerkraut to their veggie smoothie. Sauerkraut juice on its own is even sold as a digestive tonic.

One huge nutritional property of sauerkraut is that it is a surprisingly rich source of probiotics. Sauerkraut actually tops the charts for probiotic rich foods. It is said to contain more probiotics per gram than any dairy products or supplement sold over the counter. And research has been conducted to prove this shocking revelation about sauerkraut.

Research by a team led by probiotic enthusiast, Dr. Joseph M. Mercola showed that a four to six ounce serving of sauerkraut literally contained 10 trillion beneficial bacteria which is approximately equivalent to about 100 times the amount of bacteria in a bottle of high potency probiotics.[15] This shows that a 2 ounce serving of fermented sauerkraut made at home delivers approximately the same amount of probiotics contained in a bottle of 100 capsules of probiotic supplements. Which means it would take you swallowing 8 bottles of probiotics to get the same amount of supplements in a 16 ounce serving of homemade sauerkraut!

In comparison to yoghurt, for example, while 100 grams of yoghurt contains about 100 million parts of probiotics, 100 grams of sauerkraut contains a whopping 10 trillion grams of probiotics![16] "With every mouthful of sauerkraut, you're consuming billions of beneficial microbes which will be killing the pathogens in your gut driving them out and replenishing the beneficial flora in your digestive tract"- according to Dr. Natasha Campbell-McBride at the 2013 The Gluten Summit. (Plotner, 2014).

In addition to probiotics, sauerkraut also delivers several other nutrients like Vitamin A and up to 200 times more Vitamin C than the head of cabbage. You certainly have nothing to lose consuming this wonderful food.

5. Microalgae (Spirulina & Chlorella)

Some super foods that grow on the floors of the ocean are becoming increasingly popular because of their ability to increase probiotics like lactobacillus and bifidobacteria in the digestive tract. Examples include spirulina, chlorella and other edible blue-green algae. These microalgae are widely distributed in nature and similar to bacteria, not seaweed.

They have been cultivated as food for decades and are sometimes available in powder forms.[17][18] Millions of Asians, Olympic athletes and even NASA astronauts consume microalgae for the rich nutrition it supplies. Spirulina is about 65% protein and Chlorella 45% of protein. In combination, they also deliver other nutrients like carbohydrates, fiber, vitamins and minerals.

Spirulina is a safe source of nutrients which has been used for years. In addition to being nutritious, it is also known to have detoxification properties. Chlorella looks very similar to spirulina and can particularly help remove heavy metals in the body and boost liver health.[19] The rich chlorophyll content helps cleanse the digestive tract and the also contain good amounts of protein, antioxidants and vitamins that are very easy to absorb. They are also packed with energy and increase your vigor when consumed.

In recent times, the practice of introducing spirulina and chlorella into fermented milk like yoghurt to increase probiotic activity is increasingly popular. The addition of microalgae such as these can raise the viability of probiotics in fermented dairy products like yogurt.

One study showed that the addition of spirulina and chlorella in fermented milk not only increased the viability of probiotics in the product but the functional characteristic of the probiotic as well. (Beheshtipour, Mortazavian, Mohammadi, Sohrabvandi, & Khosravi-Darani, 2013) This is because these two microalgae contain a wide range of nutrients and nutraceuticals hence they are "functional foods". Functional foods simply mean foods containing health-giving additives.

Microalgae are a dense source of potent nutrition and there are several ways to incorporate them into your diet. It is said that the quantity of microalgae in contained in tiny tablet size supplement (which might be equivalent to half a teaspoon of powdered algae), can deliver the nutrition delivers the same amount of nutrition that can be derived from eating salads all day long. It can be added to smoothies, shakes, yoghurts, milk, peanut butter, sandwiches, or be chewed on its own and swallowed with water.

6. Dark Chocolate

Organic, raw, unprocessed dark chocolate has many health benefits and is even considered as a health food. Mayans even called cocoa the 'food of the gods'. Ancient Aztecs ground cocoa seeds with seasoning into a drink they thought promoted good health and their guess was correct.

Dark chocolate is often thought of as containing probiotics, but it is actually a great natural 'protector' of probiotics so it is great when combined with probiotic foods like yoghurt to preserve the good bacteria in them when we ingest them.

In Louisiana State University, researchers tested the effect of dark chocolate on stomach bacteria by comparing three different cocoa powders in a simulated human digestive process.[20] They observed that the good bacteria in the gut are able to process the flavonol compounds in the dark chocolate and also break down the dietary fiber in the dark chocolate so it can be easily absorbed.

Cocoa powder from which dark chocolate is made is rich in two flavonol compounds namely catechin and epicatechin. It also contains little dietary fiber which is fermented. The good gut bacteria are able to break down large polyphenolic polymers into smaller, anti-inflammatory molecules which are then easily absorbed in the body. [20]

Put in a simpler way, bacteria in our gut are able to break down and release the healthy nutritional content in dark chocolate.

There are several food sources that contain probiotics. The problem is that our stomach acids usually kill these organisms even before they get to the large intestine.[21] The superior trait dark chocolate has above some of these probiotic food sources is that it can deliver probiotics directly to the large intestine without being destroyed by the acidity of the secretions in the stomach walls. Dark chocolate acts as a natural protector against stomach acids and also protects against bio salts which destroy probiotics.

One study in Ghent University in Belgium revealed that dark chocolate actually protects the probiotic bacteria in the stomach and intestinal tract much better than dairy products like milk or yoghurt. The same study showed that there is a three times more percentage likelihood of probiotics surviving if it was combined with healthy dark chocolate. (Possemiers , Marzorati , Verstraete, & Van de , 2010)

With the outcome of research into dark chocolate, you cannot go wrong adding dark chocolate to your diet. It is also important you use dark chocolate with at least 70% cocoa content and no more than 3 ounces or 85 grams daily to gain valuable nutritional benefits.[22] One last thing is that most of us have become so accustomed to the taste of regular chocolate so it might take a while for our taste buds to adjust to dark chocolate. Little bites at a time will do for a start and then it can be increased with time.

7. Green Pickles

Widely available and largely taken for granted, the common pickle is a rich source of probiotics. Pickles are so easy to make if you choose not to buy the commercially available ones and they taste great.

Pickling foods is not in any way a new thing. It has been done since pre-historic times. As far back as 2030BC, it is on record that pickled cucumbers from India actually kick-started a pickling culture in Tigris Valley. Even Cleopatra was aware of the health benefits of pickles and attributed her beauty to them. (Terebelsk & Ralph, 2003) Pickles are enjoyed in many cultures throughout the world. Whole cucumbers and even chopped cucumbers are pickled. Napoleon loved pickles so much that he offered a cash prize to find a way to preserve them for longer which led to a man named Nicholas Appert to discover that immersing the glass jars used for pickling in a hot bath killed bacteria and allowed the pickles last longer.[23]

If you are buying and not making your own pickle, organic pickles that do not contain vinegar and were processed without heat are your best option to get a good dose of probiotics. Vinegar pickling i.e. immersing the green vegetable in vinegar/acetic acid significantly inhibits the growth of pathogenic microbes and yeast in the pickles.

Unfortunately, a major proportion of commercially sold pickles is made with vinegar because making pickles in this way extends the shelf life of the pickle far much longer. The exceptions to these are the half-sour pickles that are usually made in brine that has no vinegar and kept refrigerated in health food stores. They are usually more expensive in comparison to when they are made at home.

Homemade pickles fermented water, spices and brine are best. When you assemble green vegetables in a jar in your kitchen and add salt and water plus seasonings, the vegetables themselves create their own lactic acid which preserves them. These acids are a natural by-product of fermentation. This method is the traditional way of making pickles without vinegar and it is known as 'lacto-fermentation'. The sugars of greens immersed in brine draw to the surface and interact with lactic acid bacteria to produce lactic which gives the food its unique flavor and makes it still edible for a longer period. Like most fermented foods, pickles are rich probiotics.

Shorter fermenting periods of few weeks usually produce green pickles which are half sour and longer fermenting periods resulted in lighter colored pickles with more sour tastes.

Pickles can be eaten on their own as a snack, or used in sandwiches, hamburgers, hotdogs and salads. And because pickles can be eaten cold, you are certain to have the probiotics they contain when you eat them.

8. Kombucha

This is an Asian fermented tea which has been drunk for centuries and is rich in probiotics. There are several testimonials to its potency. It is said to boost immunity, help in weight loss, increase body metabolism, help in detoxification and relieves joint pain.

Kombucha is said to have originated from China before it travelled around the world to eventually attain the popularity it has today with proponents of healthy eating. Legend has it that a Japanese Emperor, Inyko, was healed by a Korean physician by the name of Kombu who gave the tea. The word 'cha' is Chinese for tea so a combination of 'Kombu' and 'cha' gave the tea its name.

Sometimes called an 'immortal health elixir', kombucha is said to give energy and immune boost, improve sleep, great for acid reflux, and other things. It is important that when if you decide to make your own kombucha, you do so in a very sanitary environments.

Kombucha is made by mixing black tea, a culture of bacteria and yeast called SCOBY[24], sugar and some kombucha in a container like a jar and allowing it to ferment for a minimum of 7 – 12 days up to a maximum of 30 days. The longer kombucha is fermented, the sourer it becomes because its sugar content is broken down. This is why some people add juice to older sour brews to make the taste more tolerable.

Health enthusiasts need to know that the sugar in kombucha cannot be avoided because it is actually what the scoby technically 'eats' in order breakdown and produce probiotics. Another new trend is replacing ordinary black tea with decaffeinated tea to reduce the caffeine content in kombucha.

Kombucha contains a lot of nutritive elements that helps balance the body's metabolism such that it can naturally heal itself that is why a lot of people feel it is a cure-all to several ailments.

One thing to note about kombucha is that it might make you worse before it makes you better. Another way to look at it is that the bad bacteria in your body will resist any good bacteria introduced to it. Kombucha doesn't agree with everyone at first and may even increase the symptoms in some diseases before it eventually gives you any relief. Starting with small quantities can help reduce this situation.

Also, pregnant women, children 10 years old and younger and people taking any blood thinners are advised not to take kombucha. About 4 to 8 ounces a day is recommended.

9. Tempeh

Tempeh is made from whole soya beans whose husk has been removed and then partially cooked then mashed and fermented with mold. During fermentation, the mold breaks down the soy mashed and binds its molecules into a cake-like form. Tempeh is widely used by vegans and vegetarians as a substitute for meat, bacon or tofu.

Its origin is said to be from Indonesia several centuries ago. Now it is eaten worldwide. Tempeh made from exclusively soya bean is popular is Indonesia. In other parts of the world, sometimes the soya bean for tempeh is also mixed with grains like millet and barley.

The fermentation process tempeh undergoes makes it easier to digest as well as to absorb. It has a good savory and nutty taste which some people describe as sweet and earthy.

It is an excellent probiotic food. It contains a lot of beneficial microorganisms particularly Rhizopus Oligosporus[25] which boosts our gut health and subsequently, the overall body. The mold or fungus used to ferment tempeh also helps produce natural antibiotics[26] which counteract the effects of certain harmful bacteria in the body.

Additionally, it is rich in other nutrients like proteins, vitamins and fiber as well as minerals like manganese, iron and other trace minerals. It's plant based protein rivals that of animal protein.

Though store-bought tempeh is convenient, it is likely to be pasteurized which means it might not contain the beneficial probiotic bacteria that are beneficial to you. And commercially sold ones usually have a slight bitter last.

Making your own tempeh[27] is encouraged but you would need to invest some time to perfect the skill particularly in regulating the temperature during the fermentation process. However once you are able to perfect the art, subsequent processes will seem like a piece of cake. And you are guaranteed to have the probiotics you need from your homemade version.

Tempeh is served in different ways. It can be boiled, fried, even grilled. In Indonesia, it is sold in almost every market and village. It can be boiled and served at home in rice or soups and it can also be found on the menu of the best fine dining restaurants. It is also good as a barbecue dish, stir fried, used as a sandwich filling substitute. Tempeh patties can be used as an alternative to beef in hamburgers. It is also used in Asian sauces. Tempeh is sometimes served raw, but the taste of raw tempeh might not agree with everyone.

10. Kimchi

Often served as an accompaniment to many meals like rice, soup, dumplings, in rolls, particularly in Korea, this Asian fermented cabbage can best be described as a spicier and slightly sour tasting variant of the sauerkraut.

Basically, cabbage is first soaked in brine to kill off any harmful bacteria inside it. After this, the cabbage is soaked in a spicy mix called gochugaru[28] then left to ferment for about 1-5 days. Sometimes the best tasting kimchi are the ones left to ferment for up to two weeks.

During this period, lacto-fermentation occurs. The lactobacillus bacteria break down the sugars in the cabbage into lactic acid leaving the cabbage with a new, sour taste. When fermented, kimchi is best preserved in the fridge.

Kimchi contains a lot of probiotics i.e. good bacteria strains. It is said that about 12 strains of lactobacillus that are able to survive in the stomach and duodenum can be found in kimchi. In addition to this, the strains of probiotics in kimchi actually adhere to the gut much better than those found in probiotic supplements (Lee, et al., 2010).

In addition, to its rich probiotic content, kimchi has been shown to have other health benefits like lowering cholesterol[29], combatting dermatitis, curbing obesity, anti-aging and many more. Being a vegetable, it is great for vegans and vegetarians.

Kimchi is easy to make and there are over a hundred different types. Some people jazz their kimchi up by adding other ingredients like a little sugar, carrots, garlic, ginger, kelp powder, seafood flavor, etc. Some people like it very hot and some mild so when you make your own kimchi, you can regulate the amount of heat by toning down or increasing the quantity of gochugaru you add.

It is advised that little quantities of kimchi should be consumed at a time. Because of its high salt content, people with high blood pressure need to consume kimchi in far lesser quantities than the average person.

11. Aged Cheese

Lately, cheese has received a lot of negative publicity particularly for having high cholesterol and promoting obesity. We are however quick to forget that certain people like the French, eat cheese much more than most of us and they have remained slimmer and had lesser cases of cardiovascular disease than the Americans.

Studies by the American Chemical Society showed that balancing out the consumption of saturated fat, physical activities, eating abundant fruits and vegetables, were extra things the French did which boosted their health. The quantity and quality of the cheese we eat also matters. Consuming cheese in moderation is important as well as consuming good brands. (Bushak, 2015)

One or two ounces of cheese a day is a good quantity to stick with. Opting for the naturally fermented cheese instead of the brands injected with bacteria by the manufacturer is best. The best type of cheese that will deliver rich amounts of probiotics are cheese made from raw, unpasteurized goat or cow milk and cheese that has aged. That said, cheese with the words 'organic', 'made from raw milk' or 'probiotic' on its label, is always your best choice to buy.

Naturally fermented cheese is loaded with lactic acid bacteria that are beneficial to our health. Cheese is actually fermented milk curds and the type of starter bacteria used, the technique and the length of fermentation time is different for various types of cheese. Because of this, different types of cheese will have different types of lactic acid bacteria.

Its low acidity and high-fat preserve makes cheese one of the perfect mediums in which healthy bacteria can grow and even be transported around the digestive system without being destroyed.

The general rule of thumb about cheese is this: any type of cheese can be rich in probiotics as long as they are not treated with heat or pasteurized after are made. That said, cheese will only deliver healthy probiotics in the body if it is not cooked before it is eaten.

Types of Cheese

Cheddars like Colby cheese, Monterey Jack, Cottage cheese
Lactococcus lactis subsp lactis
Lactococcus lactis subsp cremoris
Streptococcus thermophilus

Italian Cheese such as Parmesan, Romano, Provolone and Mozzarella
Streptococcus thermophilus
Lactobacillus delbrueckii subsp bulgaricus Lactobacillus helveticus
Lactobacillus lactis

Specialty types of cheese such as Brick, Limburger and Muenster
Lactococcus lactis subsp lactis
Lactococcus lactis subsp cremoris
Streptococcus thermophilus
Lactococcus lactis subsp biovar diacetylactis

Lactobacillus delbrueckii subsp bulgaricus Lactobacillus lactis
Lactobacillus casei subsp casei

Cheeses that have "eyes" such as Swiss, Emmental, Gouda and Edam
Lactococcus lactis subsp lactis
Lactococcus lactis subsp cremoris
Streptococcus thermophilus
Lactobacillus delbrueckii subsp bulgaricus
Lactobacillus lactis
Lactococcus lactis subsp biovar diacetylactis
Leuconostoc mesenteroides subsp cremoris
Propionibacterium shermanii

Mold ripened cheese such as Brie, Camembert, Blue, Gorgonzola and Stilton
Lactococcus lactis subsp lactis
Lactococcus lactis subsp cremoris
Lactococcus lactis subsp biovar diacetylactis
Leuconostoc mesenteroides subsp cremoris

Goat Cheese
Lactococcus lactis subsp lactis
Lactococcus lactis subsp cremoris
Lactococcus lactis subsp biovar diacetylactis
Leuconostoc mesenteroides subsp cremoris   Culled from Probiotics-LoveThatBug.com
(Rotarangi, Different Types of Cheese and the Lactic Acid Bacteria in Cheese)

Sheep Cheese
Lactococcus lactis subsp lactis
Lactococcus lactis subsp cremoris
Lactococcus lactis subsp biovar diacetylactis
Leuconostoc mesenteroides subsp cremoris

6 Other Probiotic Foods

The list of foods with probiotics does not end with the eleven that have already been mentioned. There are several more, but we will discuss 6 more probiotic foods below.

12. Olives

Olives are great snacks and one of the most nutrient dense fruits in the world. Their healthy, monounsaturated fat content delivers great health benefits to the brain, heart and waistline. They are also rich in antioxidants particularly bio phenols which are great at preventing bad cholesterol from clogging the arteries. The nutritional benefits we get from olives actually get better. Because olives are fermented, they are also rich in lactobacillus or gut-friendly bacteria.[30] Eating them is very good to gain the advantages of these healthy bacteria. Just remember that olives are usually soaked in brine so cutting down on the salt in any food they are served in would be wise to avoid excess salt consumption.

13. Wheat Grass

Most sprouted seeds and grains are actually rich in nutrition. Wheatgrass is grown from wheat seeds and contain a high level of chlorophyll and fiber. The combination of chlorophyll and fiber is great for improving colon function and essential for probiotics to thrive and keep us healthy. To get the maximum nutrition from wheatgrass, they can be juiced or dried and ground into a powder then added to shakes or smoothies.

14. Buttermilk

Buttermilk is a natural by-product of butter making process. When milk is churned, it separates into two parts: butter and whey. The whey is actually what we know as buttermilk. If made traditionally, whey is usually full of naturally occurring lactic acid bacteria which helped ferment the milk before it is churned. It has a great acidic taste which is very useful in cooking several dishes especially pancakes, pastry, pudding, or as an alternative in yoghurt dishes. However, to get the best of the healthy bacteria it contains, it should be taken cold or in cold dishes like salads, desserts or as a side dish to the main dish. Store bought buttermilk is usually pasteurized and it is skimmed milk which culture has been introduced into. Buying traditional buttermilk from health food stores is best and you should ensure it is organic and indicate on its label that it has live culture.

15. Sourdough Bread

This is a special type of bread made from a starter that is fermented for at least one day or more before it is kneaded with other ingredients to make bread. The fermentation process produces a starter that has a high concentration of beneficial bacteria. Because of this, most people believe that sourdough bread has high probiotic content as well. The problem with this assumption is that most bacteria would die from the heat required to bake bread. The claims of probiotics in sourdough bread might need more research.

16. Beer

The commercially, widely available beers that we see every day are not necessarily probiotic because even though they have been produced through a fermentation process, the yeasts and live bacteria in them are usually killed towards the end of the production process when they are pasteurized. The darker, unfiltered, unpasteurized, less common and more expensive varieties of beer usually have live cultures, but they need to be consumed in moderation to get any health benefits from them. They usually have higher alcoholic content[31] and just like wine, they can be aged because of their live cultures. The flavor is enhanced with ageing and the alcohol content also increases when it ages.

17. Natto

This is a stringy, fermented soya bean Japanese food with a distinctive pungent smell and unique flavor. It is rich in probiotics particularly bacillus subtilis formerly called bacillus antto. Natto and rice is a common breakfast serving in Japan, but it is also now added to sushi, salads and even burritos. It is a great source of plant protein and it is rich in Vitamin K. Sometimes natto is packed together with a sweet sauce which is high in fructose. The healthier way to eat natto is to forgo the sauce and opt for soy sauce instead.

Non-Dairy Probiotic Food Sources

Foods rich in probiotics seem to be main categories. They are either from dairy products or they are fermented grains or vegetables. Lactose intolerance is a growing problem worldwide, but it does not mean that anyone who suffers from lactose intolerance is at a disadvantage when it comes to probiotic foods. There are several alternatives to choose from.

Foods fermented from vegetable like pickles, sauerkraut and kimchi are great options for people who are lactose intolerant. Again, foods fermented from grains like soybeans like tempeh and miso also make great alternatives to dairy. So the problem of lactose intolerance is not really a huge issue.

Again, as said several times in this book, fermentation actually breaks down a lot of complex compounds in food and makes it tolerable for the human digestive system to digest and absorb. This includes foods that are dairy products. A food like kefir is a great example. Even though kefir is dairy based, the introduction of kefir grains into milk and the fermentation period it undergoes afterwards to produce kefir drink breaks the lactose down to a final end product that is well tolerated by even people who are lactose intolerant.

Even well aged, hard cheese with less liquid can be eaten by lactose intolerant people because the hardness actually stems from the absence of lactose which is liquid. So do try to get probiotics in good quantities into your diet even if you are lactose intolerant.

A Word About Probiotic Supplements

If all goes well and you have increased your intake of probiotic foods but for some reason, you still need to supplement your diet, it is best you know that probiotic supplements can help but not all of them will deliver the same quality or dosage of probiotics.

Avoiding enteric-coated supplements for a start is one way to ensure you get a higher quality. They cost more and might not deliver the benefit of preventing the beneficial organisms from interacting with the highly acidic digestive juices that might kill them. It is best you purchase probiotic supplements that contain a strain of organism that are resistant to stomach acids. Most of them will be well absorbed if they are taken on an empty stomach about fifteen or twenty minutes before a meal when the stomach's pH level is really at it's lowest.

Also, avoid any probiotic supplement with magnesium stearate. It is added to prevent to tablets from caking and make them mold into shape, but it does more harm than good.

Ensure you are buying from a reliable, reputable and trustworthy supplement manufacturer.

Summary & Conclusion

Raw, organic and unpasteurized food is slowly gaining popularity because of the increase in awareness of the need to eat healthily. And this trend is highly encouraging.

The benefits of probiotics to our bodies simply cannot be ignored. Probiotic rich foods are wide and varied. A good number of them can be made with food that is abundant and are quite easy to ferment. The lactobacillus bacteria which is produced from fermentation and found in probiotic food is usually different in different types of food. And every type of bacteria plays a different role. Eating a variety of different naturally fermented foods, can help us get the benefits of different probiotic bacteria.

If we cannot make our own probiotic food, and we must buy it is the store, it is best we avoid pasteurized food that is made with genetically modified raw materials and loaded with preservatives. Use of undesirable ingredients or presence of certain ingredients already is a warning signal that the beneficial bacteria and their health promoting properties we are looking for is probably not present in the food.

We must endeavor to buy organic brands from a trusted source and make a good investment into understanding how to read food labels to know exactly what is contained in the food we eat. Buying organic and buying from health food stores might be more expensive but medical treatment costs surpass any costs that may be incurred to eat right and prevent disease.

If we are preparing probiotic dishes at home, sanitary environments, minimal heat and light processing methods will ensure that we get the maximum delivery of the probiotics into our system. Wherever possible, eating probiotic foods cold or at room temperature is best as most microorganisms usually die with heat.

We must also pay attention to storing probiotic or fermented foods properly. The storage method during fermentation may differ from the storage method for storing once opened for consumption. Whilst fermentation is usually done at room temperature, the best storage for most fermented foods is usually refrigeration.

With this said, consuming probiotic rich foods should not be a one-off thing or a once-in-a-lifetime event if we truly want to get the benefits these microorganisms deliver. Eating fermented foods must become our culture. Something we do regularly.

Certain kinds of people will particularly benefit from a diet of probiotics. These are people who have been on antibiotic medication, yeast infection or overgrowth, people who have had food poisoning or digestive disturbances, people who have skin conditions like breakouts or acne, people who have mood swings and those whose immunity is generally weak. If you have experienced any of these incidents, particularly in the last one year, it is likely your probiotic level is low and you need to replenish it.

For everyone, regardless of whether you have any health condition or not, the larger/long term goal should be to fully adopt healthy eating patterns in order to maintain a healthy lifestyle. It is not enough to just introduce probiotics into our diets. While this is noble and a step in the right direction, an entire change of diet should be our bigger goal. Less sugar, salt, hydrogenated fat, carbonated drinks, processed foods, more water, fruit and vegetables, proteins, fiber, natural juices, smoothies and shakes, exercise and other healthy habits to increase the overall quality of our life. Only then would we reap huge rewards from healthy eating.

Thank you so much for downloading my book!! If you enjoyed it at all I would be forever grateful if you would leave me a review on Amazon.com

All the best!!

Endnotes

[1] 30-40 of these 400 different bacteria make up 99% of the total bacteria in our gut. (Evolve Medical Associates, 2012)

[2] This statistic refers to upper GI tract problems like acid reflux or acid indigestion (heartburn), GERD (gastroesophageal reflux disease) and ulcers. (Rafetto , Grumet, & French)

[3] (Zhong, Zhang, & Covasa, 2014)

[4] Prescription medication like antibiotics actually destroys both the good and bad bacteria in our body and it is necessary we replenish with a probiotic rich diet after taking prescription drugs.

[5] Yoghurt containing bacteria like bifidus regularis would probably be good for digestive problems like constipation. (WebMD)

[6] Study on Irritable Bowel Syndrome (O'Mahony, et al., 2005), study on diarrhea (Hempel, Newberry, Mahe, Wang, Miles, & Shanman, 2012)

[7] This story originates from the Caucasian mountains. (Coproweb)

[88] Kefir also contains a type of carbohydrate known as 'kefiran' which has antibacterial properties. (Leech, 2015)

[9] The probiotic microbes in kefir are heat sensitive hence die during pasteurization. (Gremont, 2012)

[10] Any other legume can be used as an alternative to soya beans

[11] The actual process of making miso is really much more elaborate than described in this short paragraph. (Workman, 2012)

[12] Sometimes, soya bean is added to the rice and sometimes, soya bean is used instead of rice. (Clearspring, 2013)

[13] Too much salt in the diet, spikes up the blood pressure. In addition to this, people on anti-depressant medication should avoid miso because it contains an amino acid called tyramine that can interact with certain antidepressant medications.

[14] The quantity of salt should be about two percent (2%) the weight of the cabbage prepared.

[15] This is about a hundred times the amount of bacteria in a bottle of high potency probiotic supplements (Mercola, 2013)

[16] Homemade sauerkraut will deliver this quantity of probiotics per gram. (Daily Health Post, 2014)

[17] On the side, microalgae are also an excellent source of biofuel with industrial size cultivation plants springing up all over the world.

[18] In the 1950's, the Carnegie Institute and later, the Rockefeller foundation offered huge grants to promote mass production of algae after its nutritional pedigree began to soar. It took ten years but Japan finally turned algae production into a multi-billion dollar industry. (Greenfield, 2015)

[19] A study found that mercury concentrations in the blood decreased when animals were fed chlorella. (Shim , et al., 2008)

[20] (The Alternative Daily, 2014)

[21] The presence of probiotics in the large intestine is necessary to deliver the health benefits we require from them.

[22] As suggested by Lynn Goldstein, Registered Dietitian in the You Tube Video 'Is Dark Chocolate Healthy? | HealthiNation'

[23] This hot bath method is still used till date (Rayment W.J.)

[24] SCOBY is an acronym for 'Symbiotic Culture of Bacteria and Yeast' (Laird, 2013)

[25] In addition to boosting digestive health, Rhyzopus Oligosporus also improve skin health. It is said to help with skin conditions like pimples, atopic dermatitis and cellulitis. (Amnesiana, 2013)

[26] The fermentation process produces an enzyme called phytase which helps break down phytate acid in the digestive system. Phytate acid helps increase the absorption of minerals like zinc, calcium and iron. (Amnesiana, 2013)

[27] Using organic or non-genetically modified soya beans is best and you are able to control the quality and quantity of product in your homemade version unlike what you buy in the stores.

[28] Gochugaru is a sort of dried, powdered red pepper seasoning and the ingredients for the spice mix has been kept secret for years.

[29] Two separate studies have proved kimchi's cholesterol lowering ability (Stella) (Park , Jeong , Lee , & Daily, 2013)

[30] Olives are also anti-inflammatory because they contain phenolic compounds (Oaklander, 2015)

[31] Upwards of 7% alcohol content.

Works Cited

The Alternative Daily. (2014, March 31). *Dark Chocolate and Your Gut: The Final Verdict*. Retrieved December 8, 2015, from TheAlternativeDaily.com: http://www.thealternativedaily.com/dark-chocolate-gut-final-verdict/

Amnesiana, F. (2013, September 2). *Tempeh – The Super Healthy Probiotics Food*. Retrieved December 10, 2015, from BeforeItsNews.com: http://beforeitsnews.com/health/2013/09/tempeh-the-super-healthy-probiotics-food-2503522.html

Beheshtipour, H., Mortazavian, A., Mohammadi, R., Sohrabvandi, S., & Khosravi-Darani, K. (2013). Supplementation of Spirulina platensis and Chlorella vulgaris Algae into Probiotic Fermented Milks. *Comprehensive Reviews in Food Science and Food Safety*, 144-154.

Binns, N. (2013). *Probiotics, Prebiotics and the Gut Microbiota*. Brussels, Belgium: ILSI Europe (International Life Sciences Institute).

Body Ecology Inc. (n.d.). *What is Kefir?* Retrieved December 7, 2015, from Kefir.net: http://www.kefir.net/what-is-kefir/

Bushak, L. (2015 , April 14). *List Of Healthy Foods For Gut Bacteria Expands To Include Cheese*. Retrieved December 10, 2015, from Medicaldaily.com: http://www.medicaldaily.com/list-healthy-foods-gut-bacteria-expands-include-cheese-329202

Caldwell, G. (2012, December 20). *Do Aged Cheeses Contain Probiotics?* Retrieved December 10, 2015, from GianaclisCaldwell.com: http://gianacliscaldwell.com/2012/12/20/do-aged-cheeses-contain-probiotics/

Casto, R. (2015, September 8). *What Raw Cheese Has Probiotics?* Retrieved December 10, 2015, from LiveStrong.com: http://www.livestrong.com/article/376811-what-raw-cheese-has-probiotics/

Clearspring. (2013, June 3). *Koji - The Culture Behind Japanese Food Production*. Retrieved December 8, 2015, from Clearspring.co.uk: http://www.clearspring.co.uk/blogs/news/8024723-koji-the-culture-behind-japanese-food-production

Cook, M. S. (2015). *The Probiotic Promise (Simple Steps To Heal Your Body From Inside Out)*. Philadelphia: Da Capo Press.

Coproweb. (n.d.). *Kefiranglais*. Retrieved December 7, 2015, from Coproweb.free.fr: http://coproweb.free.fr/kefiranglais.htm

Daily Health Post. (2014, July 10). *Sauerkraut Lab Results Reveal Shocking Probiotic Count…It's Even Better Than Yogurt!* Retrieved December 7, 2015, from DailyHealthPost.com: http://dailyhealthpost.com/lab-results-reveal-shocking-probiotics-count-in-sauerkraut/

Evolve Medical Associates. (2012, October 15). *Why Do I Need A Probiotic?* Retrieved December 8, 2015, from EvolveMeToday.com: http://evolvemetoday.com/blog/2012/10/15/why-do-i-need-a-probiotic

FAO & WHO. (2006). *Probiotics In Food Health And Nutritional Properties And Guidelines For Evaluation.* Rome: World Health Organisation & Food & Agriculture Organisation of the United Nations.

Gholipour, B. (2014, June 12). *Digging into Probiotics: Experts Look at Foods' Bacteria & Health Claims.* Retrieved December 10, 2015, from LiveScience.com: http://www.livescience.com/46298-the-lowdown-on-probiotics.html

Goktepe, I., Juneja, V., & Ahmedna, M. (2006). *Probiotics inFood Safet y andHuman Health.* Florida: CRC Press.

Greenfield, B. (2015, September). *How To Eat Algae (The Ultimate Guide To Fueling With Spirulina And Chlorella).* Retrieved December 8, 2015, from BenGreenfieldFitness.com: http://www.bengreenfieldfitness.com/2015/09/how-to-eat-algae/

Gremont, L. (2012, September 19). *Why I Love Kefir and What Are Kefir Grains?* Retrieved December 7, 2015, from HomemadeMommy.net: http://www.homemademommy.net/2012/09/why-i-love-kefir-and-what-are-kefir-grains.html

Grossman, K. R. (2015, May 20). *Can Probiotics Improve Your Brain?* Retrieved December 10, 2015, from WellnessMama.com: http://wellnessmama.com/54098/probiotics-improve-your-brain/

Han, E. (2013). *How To Make Easy Kimchi at Home.* Retrieved December 10, 2015, from TheKitchn.com: http://www.thekitchn.com/how-to-make-easy-kimchi-at-home-189390

Hempel, S., Newberry, S., Mahe, A., Wang, Z., Miles, J., & Shanman, R. (2012). Probiotics for the Prevention and Treatment of Antibiotic-Associated Diarrhea. *JAMA, The Journal of the American Medical Association*, 1959-1969.

Lair, C., & Sammartino, S. (2011, February). *Miso Happy Broth.* Retrieved December 8, 2015, from Cookusinterruptus.com: http://www.cookusinterruptus.com/miso-happy-broth-4136-258.html

Laird, E. (2013, March 25). *Kombucha: Myths vs. Truths*. Retrieved December 9, 2015, from PhoenixHelix.com: http://www.phoenixhelix.com/2013/03/25/kombucha-myths-vs-truths/

Lee, H., Yoon, H., Ji, Y., Kim, H., Park, H., Lee, J., et al. (2010). Functional Properties Of Lactobacillus Strains Isolated From Kimchi. *International Journal of Food Microbiology*, 155 - 161.

Leech, J. (2015, March 27). *What is Kefir and Why Is It So Good for You?* Retrieved December 7, 2015, from Ecowatch.com: http://ecowatch.com/2015/03/27/health-benefits-kefir/

Marie, J. (2015, September 23). *Which Probiotics Does Miso Contain?* Retrieved December 8, 2015, from Livestrong.com: http://www.livestrong.com/article/320105-what-probiotics-does-miso-contain/

Mercola, D. J. (2013, December 29). *Fermenting Foods—One of the Easiest and Most Creative Aspects of Making Food from Scratch*. Retrieved December 7, 2015, from Mercola.com: http://articles.mercola.com/sites/articles/archive/2013/12/29/sandor-katz-on-fermented-foods.aspx

Michaelis, K. (2008, December 13). *Kombucha Health Benefits*. Retrieved December 12, 2015, from FoodRenegade.com: http://www.foodrenegade.com/kombucha-health-benefits/

Narins, E. (2013, May 29). *The Best Yoghurt For You*. Retrieved December 8, 2015, from WomensHealthMag.com: http://www.womenshealthmag.com/food/the-best-yogurt-for-you

Oaklander, M. (2015, July 16). *Should I Eat Olives?* Retrieved December 11, 2015, from TIme.com: http://time.com/3946177/olives-nutrition-probiotics/

O'Mahony, L., McCarthy, J., Kelly, P., Hurley, G., Luo, F., Chen, K., et al. (2005). Lactobacillus and bifidobacterium in irritable bowel syndrome: symptom responses and relationship to cytokine profiles. *Gastroenterology*, 541-551.

Park, K., Jeong , J., Lee , Y., & Daily, J. (2013). Health Benefits of Kimchi (Korean Fermented Vegetables) As A Probiotic Food. *Journal of Medicinal Food*, 6 - 20.

Plotner, B. (2014, June 21). *Sauerkraut Test Divulges Shocking Probiotic Count*. Retrieved December 7, 2015, from Nourishingplot.com: http://nourishingplot.com/2014/06/21/sauerkraut-test-divulges-shocking-probiotic-count/

Possemiers , S., Marzorati , M., Verstraete, W., & Van de , W. (2010, June 30). *Bacteria And Chocolate: A Successful Combination For Probiotic Delivery*. (Laboratory of Microbial Ecology and Technology (LabMET), Ghent University, Coupure Links

653, B-9000 Ghent, Belgium) Retrieved December 8, 2015, from NCBI.nlm.nih.gov: http://www.ncbi.nlm.nih.gov/pubmed/20452073

Probiotic Help. (n.d.). *What Is Tempeh?* Retrieved December 10, 2015, from Probiotics-Help.com: http://www.probiotics-help.com/what-is-tempeh.html

Rafetto , M., Grumet, T., & French, G. (n.d.). *Effects Of Caffeine And Coffee On Heartburn, Acid Reflux, Ulcers And GERD: Effects Of Caffeine And Coffee On Heartburn, Acid Reflux, Ulcers And GERD.* Retrieved December 8, 2015 , from Healthy.net: http://www.healthy.net/Health/Article/Effects_of_Caffeine_and_Coffee_on_Heartburn_Acid_Reflux_Ulcers_and_GERD/2396

Rayment W.J. (n.d.). *Pickle History.* Retrieved December 9, 2015, from InDepthInfo.com: http://www.indepthinfo.com/pickles/history.htm

Rotarangi, D. (n.d.). *Different Types of Cheese and the Lactic Acid Bacteria in Cheese.* Retrieved December 10, 2015, from Probiotics-LoveThatBug.com: http://www.probiotics-lovethatbug.com/types-of-cheese.html

Rotarangi, D. (n.d.). *What Is A Healthy Cheese.* Retrieved December 10, 2015, from Probiotics-LoveThatBug.com: http://www.probiotics-lovethatbug.com/healthy-cheese.html

Rotarangi, D. (n.d.). *What Is Probiotic Cheese.* Retrieved December 10, 2015, from Probiotics-LoveThatBug.com: http://www.probiotics-lovethatbug.com/what-is-probiotic-cheese.html

Shim , J., Shin, H., Han, J., Park , H., Lim, B., Chung , K., et al. (2008). Protective effects of Chlorella vulgaris on liver toxicity in cadmium-administered rats. *Journal of Medicinal Food*, 479-485.

Stella. (n.d.). *Probiotics or Cultured Food: Which is Better?* Retrieved December 10, 2015, from Stellametsovas.com: http://stellametsovas.com/probiotics-or-cultured-food-which-is-better/

Taylor, J., & Mitchell, D. (2007). *The Wonder of Probiotics.* New York: St. Martin's Press.

Terebelsk, D., & Ralph, N. (2003). *Pickle History Timeline.* Retrieved December 9, 2015, from NYFoodMuseum.org: http://www.nyfoodmuseum.org/_ptime.htm

The Conscious Life. (2010, February 27). *Top Probiotic Foods You Are Not Eating.* Retrieved December 10, 2015, from TheConsciousLife.com: http://theconsciouslife.com/top-probiotic-foods.htm

The University of Dakota Dining Services. (n.d.). *Prebiotics/Probiotics.* Retrieved December 6, 2015, from UND.edu: https://und.edu/student-life/dining/_files/docs/fact-sheets/probiotics.pdf

Thompson, J. P. (2012). *What You Need To Know About Probiotics.* Caramal Publishing.

WebMD. (n.d.). *10 Tips for Buying and Eating Yogurt.* Retrieved December 8, 2015, from WebMD.com: http://www.webmd.com/diet/benefits-of-yogurt?page=4

Workman, D. (2012, February 4). *Making Miso.* Retrieved December 8, 2015, from PermacultureNews.org: http://permaculturenews.org/2012/02/04/making-miso/

Zhong, L., Zhang, X., & Covasa, M. (2014). Emerging Roles of Lactic Acid Bacteria In Protection Against Colorectal Cancer. *World Journal of Gastroenterology*, 1-10.

www.ingramcontent.com/pod-product-compliance
Lightning Source LLC
Chambersburg PA
CBHW071557170526
45166CB00004B/1707